This book was compiled
with the A.I assistance

Dedication

I hope this helps all of my wonderful readers achieve all their goals in their business. And I would like to thank my wonderful wife for all of her continued support in all my ventures.

May 7 2023

Contents

Introduction

Living with Rheumatoid Arthritis can be an invisible battle that many individuals face every day. For those who do not understand the complexities of this condition, it can be difficult to empathize with the pain, fatigue, and emotional turmoil that accompany it. This book aims to provide insight and information into navigating life with Rheumatoid Arthritis. In this book, you will find comprehensive information about the symptoms, diagnosis, and treatments available for Rheumatoid Arthritis. You will also learn about the emotional impact that this condition can have on individuals, and the coping strategies that can be adopted to manage and overcome these challenges. Living with Rheumatoid Arthritis can present many obstacles, but it is possible to maintain a fulfilling and happy life despite the difficulties. This book will provide you with valuable insights and tools for living a full life with Rheumatoid Arthritis. Coming up next in Chapter 2, we'll delve into what Rheumatoid Arthritis is and what the symptoms are.

Chapter 2: What is Rheumatoid Arthritis?

Rheumatoid arthritis (RA) is a chronic autoimmune disorder that primarily affects the joints. In this condition, the immune system mistakes the body's own healthy tissues as foreign invaders and attacks them, resulting in inflammation, pain, stiffness, and swelling in the joints. Unlike other types of arthritis, such as osteoarthritis (which is caused by wear and tear on the joints), RA can affect people of all ages and genders. While the exact cause of RA is still unknown, researchers believe that genetic, environmental, and hormonal factors may all play a role. RA typically begins in the smaller joints of the hands and feet, before spreading to other joints such as the wrists, elbows, shoulders, hips, knees, and ankles. Symptoms of RA can vary in severity and frequency and may include:

Joint symptoms:

- Pain and tenderness
- Stiffness, especially in the morning or after sitting for a long time
- Swelling and warmth
- Redness and discoloration
- Difficulty moving the joint or performing daily activities like grasping or holding items

Non-joint symptoms:

- Fatigue
- Fever
- Weight loss
- Anemia (low red blood cell count)
- Eye inflammation, dryness, or sensitivity to light
- Loss of appetite

If you are experiencing any of these symptoms, it is important to see your doctor as soon as possible for an accurate diagnosis and appropriate treatment. Early intervention can help prevent joint damage and disability associated with RA. In the next chapter, we will discuss the different methods of diagnosing RA and how to recognize the signs and symptoms.

Chapter 3: Symptoms and Diagnosis of Rheumatoid Arthritis

Rheumatoid arthritis (RA) is a chronic autoimmune disease that affects over 1.3 million people in the United States. It causes inflammation and pain in the joints, resulting in stiffness and difficulty moving. Knowing the symptoms and getting an accurate diagnosis is crucial in managing this condition.

SYMPTOMS OF RHEUMATOID ARTHRITIS

RA affects each person differently, but there are common symptoms that many people experience. These include:

Joint Pain and Stiffness

Pain and stiffness in the joints are the most common symptoms of RA. They are often worst in the morning or after periods of inactivity, and usually affect the hands, feet, wrists, and ankles. As the condition progresses, pain and stiffness can become constant and affect other joints in the body.

Fatigue

Many people with RA experience persistent fatigue. They may feel tired even after a full night's sleep or after minimal activity.

Swelling and Inflammation

RA causes inflammation in the joints, resulting in swelling, tenderness, and warmth around the affected area. This can lead to deformities in the joints over time if left untreated.

Fever and Weight Loss

Some people with RA may also experience fever and weight loss, although these symptoms are less common.

DIAGNOSIS OF RHEUMATOID ARTHRITIS

Early diagnosis and treatment of RA is important to prevent joint damage and deformity. A rheumatologist is a doctor who specializes in the treatment of autoimmune disorders and can help diagnose RA. The diagnosis of RA is based on a combination of symptoms, physical examination, and laboratory tests. The doctor will examine the joints for signs of swelling and inflammation and ask about your medical history and symptoms. Blood tests can also help diagnose RA. The rheumatoid factor (RF) is a blood test that is positive in about 80% of people with RA. Anti-cyclic citrullinated peptide (anti-CCP) is another blood test that is specific for RA and can indicate the severity of the disease. Imaging tests such as X-rays, ultrasounds, and magnetic resonance imaging (MRI) may also be used to detect joint damage and monitor disease progression.

The Bottom Line

Symptoms of RA can vary from person to person, but joint pain and stiffness are the most common. Early diagnosis and treatment are essential in managing the disease, and a rheumatologist can help diagnose and develop a treatment plan to improve quality of life. If you are experiencing joint pain, stiffness, or any of the symptoms listed above, make an appointment with your healthcare provider as soon as possible.

Chapter 4: Invisible Battles: The Emotional Impact of Rheumatoid Arthritis

Living with rheumatoid arthritis is a constant challenge. Not just physically, but emotionally as well. As a chronic condition, it never goes away, and it can be a constant source of frustration for people who live with it. Flare-ups can be unexpected and debilitating, and they can cause people to feel apprehensive about making plans or having a normal life. This can have a significant emotional impact on those with rheumatoid arthritis. In this chapter, we'll discuss some of the emotional challenges that come with living with this condition, and some strategies for managing those challenges.

RHEUMATOID ARTHRITIS AND MENTAL HEALTH

It's common for people with chronic conditions to experience mental health challenges such as anxiety and depression. Studies have shown that people with rheumatoid arthritis are at increased risk for depression and anxiety. This isn't surprising. Chronic pain and disability can be incredibly challenging to manage, and it can lead to feelings of helplessness, hopelessness, and frustration. It's also common for people with rheumatoid arthritis to experience social isolation, which can compound feelings of loneliness and depression.

COPING STRATEGIES

It's important for people with rheumatoid arthritis to find healthy ways to cope with the emotional impact of their condition.

Some strategies that may be helpful include:

1. Support Groups

Connecting with others who are going through similar experiences can be incredibly powerful. Many communities have support groups for people with rheumatoid arthritis, and there may also be online support groups that can be accessed from anywhere.

2. Therapy

Seeing a therapist can be incredibly helpful for people who are struggling with the emotional impact of rheumatoid arthritis. A therapist can help people develop coping strategies, work through difficult emotions, and manage symptoms of depression and anxiety.

3. Exercise

Exercise can be a great mood booster and can help manage symptoms of depression and anxiety. It's important for people with rheumatoid arthritis to find exercises that work for their bodies, which may mean low-impact activities such as swimming or yoga.

4. Self-Care

It's important to take care of oneself when dealing with the emotional impact of rheumatoid arthritis. This may mean setting boundaries, getting enough sleep, practicing relaxation techniques, or even just taking time for oneself to do something enjoyable.

CONCLUSION

The emotional impact of rheumatoid arthritis can be just as challenging as the physical impact. It's important for people with this condition to find healthy ways to cope, whether that means seeking support from others, seeing a therapist, or practicing self-care strategies. By taking care of oneself emotionally, people with rheumatoid arthritis can improve their overall quality of life and learn to triumph over the invisible battles associated with their condition.

Chapter 5: Treatments and Medications for Rheumatoid Arthritis

Rheumatoid Arthritis (RA) is a chronic autoimmune disease that causes inflammation in various joints of the body. While there is no cure for RA, there are several treatments and medications to help alleviate pain, reduce inflammation, and slow down joint damage.

TREATMENTS FOR RHEUMATOID ARTHRITIS

The treatment for RA aims to relieve symptoms, suppress inflammation, and prevent further joint damage. The following are some of the commonly used treatments for RA:

Nonsteroidal Anti-Inflammatory Drugs (NSAIDs)

NSAIDs can be used to relieve pain and inflammation caused by RA. They work by reducing the production of prostaglandins, which are hormone-like substances that cause pain and inflammation in the body. Some of the common NSAIDs used to treat RA include ibuprofen, aspirin, and naproxen.

Disease-Modifying Antirheumatic Drugs (DMARDs)

DMARDs are used to suppress the immune system and prevent further joint damage caused by RA. They work by altering the immune system's response to reduce inflammation. Some of the common

DMARDs used to treat RA include methotrexate, sulfasalazine, and hydroxychloroquine.

Biologic Response Modifiers (BRMs)

BRMs are genetically engineered medications that target specific proteins in the immune system to reduce inflammation caused by RA. Some of the common BRMs used to treat RA include etanercept, infliximab, and adalimumab.

Corticosteroids

Corticosteroids or steroids are a type of medication that reduces inflammation by suppressing the immune system. They can be used alone or in combination with other drugs to control pain, swelling, and stiffness caused by RA. Some of the common steroids used to treat RA include prednisone and methylprednisolone.

MEDICATIONS FOR RHEUMATOID ARTHRITIS

Apart from the above treatments, medications can also be used to manage the symptoms of RA. Some of the common medications used to treat RA include:

Pain Relievers

Pain relievers can be used to reduce the pain caused by RA. Some of the common pain relievers used to treat RA include acetaminophen and tramadol.

Topical Analgesics

Topical analgesics can be applied to the skin to relieve pain caused by RA. Some of the common topical analgesics used to treat RA include gels and creams that contain capsaicin.

Joint Injections

Joint injections can be used to relieve pain and inflammation caused by RA. They can be given directly into the affected joint to provide fast, targeted relief. Some of the common joint injections used to treat RA include corticosteroids and hyaluronic acid.

Vitamins and Supplements

Certain vitamins and supplements can be used to manage the symptoms of RA. Some of the common vitamins and supplements used to treat RA include vitamin D, omega-3 fatty acids, and glucosamine. In conclusion, there are several treatments and medications available to manage the symptoms of RA. It's essential to work closely with a healthcare professional to determine the most suitable treatment plan for you. By following a comprehensive treatment plan, people with RA can manage their symptoms, improve their quality of life, and reduce the impact of the disease on their daily lives.

Chapter 6: The Importance of Diet and Exercise for Managing Rheumatoid Arthritis

Rheumatoid arthritis (RA) is an autoimmune disease that causes inflammation in the joints, leading to pain, stiffness, and limited mobility. Although RA cannot be cured, proper management can help alleviate its symptoms and slow its progression. In addition to medications and other therapies, lifestyle changes such as diet and exercise play a crucial role in managing RA.

DIETARY CONSIDERATIONS FOR RA PATIENTS

A balanced and nutritious diet is essential for everyone, but it is particularly important for those with RA. While no specific diet has been proven to cure or treat RA, there are certain foods that can help alleviate inflammation, reduce pain, and improve overall health.

Anti-Inflammatory Foods

Some foods have anti-inflammatory properties, which can help reduce inflammation and relieve pain in RA patients. Examples of such foods include fatty fish (such as salmon and tuna), nuts (such as almonds and walnuts), fruits (such as blueberries and cherries), vegetables (such as broccoli and spinach), and whole grains (such as brown rice and quinoa).

Vitamin D and Calcium

Vitamin D and calcium are essential for maintaining strong bones, which is especially important for people with RA. RA patients are at increased risk for osteoporosis, a condition in which bones become brittle and fragile. Foods rich in vitamin D and calcium include dairy products, leafy greens (such as kale and collard greens), and fortified cereals and juices.

Weight Management

Maintaining a healthy weight is crucial for RA patients, as excess weight puts extra stress on the joints. In addition, adipose tissue (fat) produces chemicals that can promote inflammation in the body, aggravating RA symptoms. A balanced diet that includes lean protein, fruits, vegetables, and whole grains can help RA patients achieve and maintain a healthy weight.

EXERCISE AND RA

Although it may seem counterintuitive, exercise is actually beneficial for people with RA. Exercise helps maintain joint flexibility, reduce inflammation, improve muscle strength and endurance, and enhance overall well-being. However, it is important for RA patients to engage in the right types of exercise, at the right intensity and frequency, in order to avoid further joint damage and pain.

Low-Impact Exercises

Low-impact exercises such as walking, cycling, swimming, and yoga are ideal for RA patients, as they provide cardiovascular benefits without putting excessive stress on the joints. Strength training exercises that target specific muscle groups can also help improve joint stability and function.

Stretching and Range of Motion Exercises

Stretching and range of motion exercises are important for maintaining joint flexibility and preventing stiffness. These exercises can be done at home, and should be performed daily for best results.

Pacing and Rest

RA patients should avoid overexertion and fatigue, as these can exacerbate joint pain and inflammation. Pacing oneself during exercise, and taking frequent breaks when needed, can help prevent joint damage and optimize the benefits of exercise. In summary, diet and exercise are important components of a holistic approach to managing RA. By eating a balanced, nutritious diet rich in anti-inflammatory foods, maintaining a healthy weight, and engaging in the right types of low-impact exercise and stretching, RA patients can improve joint function and mobility, reduce pain and inflammation, and enhance overall quality of life.

Chapter 7: Coping Strategies for Living with Rheumatoid Arthritis

Rheumatoid arthritis is a chronic illness that can take a toll on your physical and mental well-being. Coping strategies can help you manage the challenges of living with this condition. In this chapter, we will explore some effective coping strategies that can help you live a happier and healthier life with rheumatoid arthritis.

MIND-BODY TECHNIQUES

Mind-body techniques are a collection of practices that integrate the mind and body to promote relaxation and well-being. These techniques can help reduce stress, anxiety, and pain associated with rheumatoid arthritis. Popular mind-body techniques include:

Meditation

Meditation is a mental practice that involves focusing your attention on a word, phrase, or sound with the goal of achieving a calm and relaxed state of mind. Practicing meditation regularly can help reduce stress and anxiety and promote relaxation.

Yoga

Yoga is a physical practice that involves a series of postures, breathing exercises, and meditation. Practicing yoga regularly can help improve flexibility, balance, and strength, as well as reduce stress and anxiety.

COGNITIVE-BEHAVIORAL THERAPY

Cognitive-behavioral therapy (CBT) is a form of talk therapy that helps individuals manage their thoughts, emotions, and behaviors. CBT can help individuals with rheumatoid arthritis learn how to identify and challenge negative thoughts and behaviors that contribute to their physical and emotional pain.

PHYSICAL ACTIVITY

Physical activity, such as exercise or walking, can help improve joint flexibility, reduce pain and inflammation, and increase energy levels. Exercise can also help boost mood and reduce stress and anxiety associated with rheumatoid arthritis.

ASSISTIVE DEVICES

Assistive devices, such as canes, walkers, or braces, can help individuals with rheumatoid arthritis perform daily activities with less pain and discomfort. Using assistive devices can also help reduce the risk of falls and injuries.

SOCIAL SUPPORT

Social support from friends, family members, or support groups can help individuals with rheumatoid arthritis feel less isolated and alone. Support from others can also provide emotional and practical assistance to help manage the challenges of living with this condition.

CONCLUSION

Living with rheumatoid arthritis can be challenging, but coping strategies can help minimize the impact of this condition on your life. Mind-body techniques, cognitive-behavioral therapy, physical activity, assistive devices, and social support are all effective coping strategies to help manage the physical and emotional challenges of living with rheumatoid arthritis. Experiment with different coping strategies to find what works best for you, and don't be afraid to seek help and support when needed.

Support Networks for People with Rheumatoid Arthritis

Living with rheumatoid arthritis can be challenging, but the burden can be made lighter by building a strong support network. A support network can provide emotional and practical support, advice, and encouragement. This chapter will discuss the importance of support networks for people with rheumatoid arthritis and how to build one.

WHY SUPPORT NETWORKS ARE ESSENTIAL FOR PEOPLE WITH RHEUMATOID ARTHRITIS

Dealing with a chronic condition like rheumatoid arthritis can take a toll on a person's mental and emotional health. Support networks can provide a safe space for people with rheumatoid arthritis to share their feelings and experiences with people who understand what they're going through. Being part of a support network can also help to reduce feelings of loneliness and isolation that can come with having a chronic condition. Additionally, a support network can provide practical help with daily tasks such as grocery shopping, housework, and transportation to medical appointments. Friends, family, and healthcare providers can also be involved in making decisions about treatment options, which can help to ensure that the person with rheumatoid arthritis is receiving the best possible care.

BUILDING A SUPPORT NETWORK

Building a support network takes time and effort, but it's worth it in the end. Here are some tips for building a strong support network:

1. Reach Out to Friends and Family

The first step in building a support network is to reach out to friends and family. Let them know about your condition and how it affects you. Be honest about your feelings and needs. You might be surprised at how willing people are to help.

2. Join a Support Group

Support groups are a great way to connect with other people who have rheumatoid arthritis. They provide a safe and supportive environment for people to share their experiences and learn from others. Consider joining an in-person or online support group.

3. Talk to Your Healthcare Providers

Your healthcare providers are a valuable part of your support network. They can provide advice, guidance, and support. Be open and honest with them about how you're feeling and what your needs are.

4. Consider Professional Counseling

Living with rheumatoid arthritis can be stressful and overwhelming. Professional counseling can help you to cope with the emotional and mental challenges that come with having a chronic condition.

CONCLUSION

Building a support network is an essential part of managing rheumatoid arthritis. It can provide emotional and practical support, reduce feelings of loneliness and isolation, and help with decision-making about treatment options. Reach out to friends and family, join a support group, talk to your healthcare providers, and consider professional counseling to build a strong and supportive network.

Chapter 9: Living a Full Life with Rheumatoid Arthritis: Stories of Inspiration

INTRODUCTION

When you're living with rheumatoid arthritis, it can be difficult to imagine a future where you're able to do the things you love without pain or discomfort. But the truth is, there are countless people with RA who are living proof that it's possible to lead a full, active life despite the challenges they face every day. In this chapter, we'll share inspiring stories from those who have learned to navigate life with rheumatoid arthritis, offering hope and encouragement to anyone struggling with this chronic illness.

OVERCOMING THE ODDS: STORIES OF TRIUMPH

Living with RA can be a daunting prospect, and it's easy to feel like your world is shrinking as the disease progresses. But for some, that sense of loss and limitation is just the fuel they need to push themselves even further. Take, for example, John, a former marathon runner who was diagnosed with RA in his early 30s. After many years of struggling to keep up with his passion for running, he decided to try a new approach: triathlons. Despite the added challenges of swimming and biking, John found that the variation and cross-training actually helped him manage his symptoms. Today, he's completed multiple Ironman races and even holds a few age-group records. Or consider Jennifer, a professional dancer who feared she would never perform again after her diagnosis. But instead of giving up on her dream, she worked with her healthcare team to find creative ways to modify her routines and develop new techniques that put less strain on her joints. Through hard work and persistence, Jennifer has continued to dance professionally for more than a decade, even choreographing her own productions. These stories, and so many more like them, are a reminder that with determination and a positive attitude, you can overcome even the greatest odds.

ADAPTING TO NEW REALITIES: STORIES OF RESILIENCE

Of course, not everyone with RA will be able to continue pursuing their passions in the same way they always have. For some, adapting to life with chronic illness means learning to find new sources of joy and meaning. Consider Tom, a former carpenter who had to retire early due to debilitating hand and wrist pain. Despite the loss of his career, he discovered a new talent in painting, taking up watercolors and finding great satisfaction in creating landscapes and seascapes from his backyard. Painting gave

Tom a new sense of purpose and helped him find joy in life, even amid the challenges of his illness. Likewise, Angie, a busy mother of three, had to learn to scale back her expectations and prioritize self-care after her RA diagnosis. By taking things one day at a time and focusing on what really mattered most, Angie found that she could still be the loving, involved parent she wanted to be, even if that meant letting go of some of her outside commitments. Today, she cherishes the moments she spends with her kids and finds strength in knowing that she's doing what's best for her health. These stories remind us that it's possible to find happiness and fulfillment in all sorts of unexpected places, even when life doesn't go as planned.

LESSONS LEARNED: ADVICE FROM THOSE WHO HAVE BEEN THERE

For anyone struggling with RA, it can be incredibly helpful to hear from others who have gone through similar experiences. Here are some words of wisdom from those who have learned to navigate life with rheumatoid arthritis: -"Take things one day at a time. Some days will be better than others, but the key is to keep going and not give up." -Emily, 37 -"Don't be afraid to ask for help when you need it. Friends and family are there to support you." -Ben, 46 -"Find ways to stay active that work for you. It might not be the same as before, but that doesn't mean you can't stay fit and healthy." -Jessica, 52 -"Remember to be kind to yourself. It's OK to take things slower and make adjustments to your life as needed." -Adam, 30 These insights remind us that we are not alone in our struggles, and that there is always hope for a brighter future.

CONCLUSION: LIVING A FULL LIFE WITH RHEUMATOID ARTHRITIS

Living with rheumatoid arthritis can be challenging, but it's important to remember that it's not the end of the road. With the right attitude, support, and mindset, it's possible to continue pursuing the things you love and finding happiness in all sorts of unexpected places. We hope these stories have inspired you to keep pushing forward and living a full life, no matter what challenges you may face.

Subchapter 1: The Challenges of Parenting with Rheumatoid Arthritis

Rheumatoid Arthritis can be a daunting diagnosis for anyone, but for parents, its impact can be even more overwhelming. Navigating the challenges of parenting while battling the daily pain that comes with Rheumatoid Arthritis can be an uphill battle, but it is one that many parents with the condition have learned to manage with confidence. One significant challenge that parents with Rheumatoid Arthritis face is the impact the condition can have on their ability to physically care for their children.

Simple tasks such as picking up a baby, carrying a toddler, or even playing with children can become incredibly difficult when experiencing the chronic pain and inflammation of Rheumatoid Arthritis. Another difficulty that Rheumatoid Arthritis can bring to parenting is the guilt that can arise from not being able to participate in certain activities or duties due to the condition's limitations. It's important for parents to remember that they are still capable of providing love and support to their children, even if it may look different from what they are used to. In addition, managing Rheumatoid Arthritis while raising children can require extra planning and accommodations. For example, parents may need to schedule certain activities or events around their medication schedules or arrange for extra help with childcare during times of increased pain or fatigue. Despite the many challenges that Rheumatoid Arthritis can bring to parenting, it's essential to stay hopeful and seek out support. Joining a support group specific to parenting with Rheumatoid Arthritis can be an excellent way to connect with others facing similar challenges and gain advice and insight from those who have already navigated the ups and downs of raising children with the condition. The key to success in parenting with Rheumatoid Arthritis is to be kind and patient with oneself. Remember that living with the condition is challenging, but with the right support and resources, it is possible to thrive.

WORKING WITH RHEUMATOID ARTHRITIS

Rheumatoid arthritis can affect your ability to work, particularly if your job involves physical labor. However, many people with this condition can continue to work by making some adjustments to their work environment and daily routine.

Talking to Your Employer

If you have rheumatoid arthritis, it's important to communicate with your employer about your condition. You may qualify for accommodations under the Americans with Disabilities Act (ADA). Accommodations can include:

- Modifications to your work schedule or hours
- Assistive devices, such as ergonomic keyboards or chairs
- Flexible breaks or work-from-home options
- Reassignment to a less physically demanding role

Your employer may also be able to help you make adjustments to your work environment, such as providing a more supportive chair or a workstation that is adapted to your needs.

Managing Your Symptoms at Work

In addition to making changes to your work environment, there are several things you can do to manage your symptoms while at work. These include:

- Taking regular breaks to move around and stretch
- Using heat or cold therapy to manage pain and stiffness
- Keeping your workspace organized and avoiding clutter
- Using assistive tools, such as a grip or jar opener, to make tasks easier

It's also important to talk to your healthcare provider about any medications or treatments that may help you manage your symptoms at work. They may be able to recommend pain management strategies or other treatments that can help you remain productive on the job.

Self-Care Strategies for Working with Rheumatoid Arthritis

In addition to making adjustments to your work environment and managing your symptoms, practicing self-care can also help you stay productive at work. Some strategies you can try include:

- Eating a healthy diet that is rich in anti-inflammatory foods
- Getting regular exercise, such as yoga or swimming
- Making time for rest and relaxation, such as taking a warm bath or meditating
- Getting enough sleep each night

By taking care of yourself and managing your symptoms, you can continue to work and pursue your career while living with rheumatoid arthritis. Remember to take things one day at a time and be kind to yourself as you navigate this condition.

Traveling with Rheumatoid Arthritis

Living with Rheumatoid Arthritis can often be challenging, especially when it comes to traveling. However, with a few simple adjustments and precautions, people with Rheumatoid Arthritis can still enjoy traveling without exacerbating their symptoms.

PREPARATION

Planning ahead is key when traveling with Rheumatoid Arthritis. Here are some important tips to keep in mind:

1. Consult with Your Doctor

Before traveling, it's vital to discuss your plans with your doctor. Your doctor may recommend specific medications or treatments for your trip, or may suggest scheduling appointments with local doctors at your destination.

2. Pack Smart

When packing for your trip, pack light and only bring the essentials to avoid overstressing your joints. Consider investing in a suitcase with wheels or a backpack to make traveling easier. Additionally, pack heat or cold pads for sore joints, extra medications, and any assistive devices you may need, like walking canes.

3. Research Your Destination

Research your destination before the trip to determine factors that may impact your Rheumatoid Arthritis, such as climate or terrain. Consider booking accessible accommodations or requesting a wheelchair or scooter rental if needed.

ON THE FLIGHT

Air travel can be particularly challenging for people with Rheumatoid Arthritis because of long periods of sitting and reduced ability to move around. Here are some tips to make air travel more comfortable:

1. Request Special Accommodations

At check-in, notify the airline of any special accommodations you may need, such as seating arrangements. Some airlines may offer extra legroom or assistive devices like a neck pillow or blanket.

2. Move Regularly

During the flight, exercise your legs by doing simple ankle and foot rotations, or consider taking short walks up and down the aisle when possible.

3. Stay Hydrated and Comfortable

Drink plenty of water to stay hydrated and avoid alcohol or caffeine, which may worsen inflammation and dehydration.

Dress comfortably, in loose-fitting clothes that won't restrict movement.

AT YOUR DESTINATION

Once you arrive at your destination, it's important to take care of your body. Here are some tips to stay comfortable during your trip:

1. Pace Yourself

It's easy to get caught up in the excitement of traveling, but it's crucial to pace yourself and avoid overexerting yourself. Plan rest breaks throughout the day and take time to relax and recharge.

2. Stay Active

Despite the temptation to relax, it's important to stay active while traveling to keep your joints from stiffening. Consider taking short walks or doing gentle stretches throughout your trip.

3. Stick to Your Medication Schedule

Traveling can disrupt your daily routine, but it's important to stick to your medication schedule to manage your Rheumatoid Arthritis symptoms. Set reminders on your phone or watch to ensure you don't miss a dose. In conclusion, traveling with Rheumatoid Arthritis may seem daunting, but with the right preparation and mindset, it can still be an enjoyable and fulfilling experience. Remember to listen to your body and take care of yourself throughout your trip.

Subchapter 4: Maintaining Relationships with Rheumatoid Arthritis

Living with rheumatoid arthritis can be a challenge, not just physically, but also socially and emotionally. Maintaining relationships with others can be especially difficult when you are dealing with chronic pain and fatigue. Here are some tips for managing your relationships while living with rheumatoid arthritis:

COMMUNICATE WITH YOUR LOVED ONES:

It's important to communicate with your loved ones honestly about how you are feeling. Let them know that you may need to take breaks or that certain activities may be difficult for you. Communication is key to maintaining strong relationships with your loved ones.

SEEK SUPPORT:

Joining a support group or seeking counseling can also be helpful in managing your relationships. Support groups can provide a safe space to discuss your condition with others who understand what you are going through. A counselor can also help you learn coping strategies and provide emotional support.

SET BOUNDARIES:

Setting boundaries can be difficult, but it is important to set limits for yourself to avoid overexertion. Communicate to your loved ones when you need to take a break or when certain activities may be too challenging for you. Remember that it's okay to say no sometimes.

FIND WAYS TO STAY CONNECTED:

While physical activities may be more challenging, finding new ways to stay connected with your loved ones can be fun and fulfilling. For example, you can plan virtual game nights, movie nights, or simply chat regularly on the phone or through social media platforms.

BE PATIENT WITH YOURSELF:

Living with rheumatoid arthritis can be frustrating, but remember to be patient with yourself and with your loved ones. It may take time for them to fully understand your condition and its impact on your life. Be open to educating them about your condition and strive to maintain positive and healthy relationships. Living with rheumatoid arthritis can be challenging, but it's important to remember that maintaining strong relationships with your loved ones is possible. Communication, support, setting boundaries, finding new ways to connect, and being patient with yourself are all key to managing your relationships and living a fulfilling life.

Chapter 10: Research and Future Directions in Rheumatoid Arthritis Management

Rheumatoid arthritis (RA) is a chronic autoimmune disorder that affects various joints in the body. It causes inflammation in the lining of the joints, which leads to painful swelling, stiffness, and eventually joint damage. While it is a manageable disease, there is still no cure for RA. However, ongoing research is exploring new treatments to alleviate symptoms and improve the quality of life for those living with RA.

THE LATEST RESEARCH IN RHEUMATOID ARTHRITIS

In recent years, researchers have made significant advances in the development of new therapies for RA. For example, a class of drugs called biologics has been developed that specifically targets cells of the immune system that are involved in the inflammation process. Some of these drugs include adalimumab, infliximab, and etanercept. Other drugs being explored in clinical trials include JAK inhibitors, which target a specific protein in the immune system that triggers inflammation. Researchers are also looking into stem cell therapy, which involves using stem cells to repair damaged joints.

PERSONALIZED MEDICINE FOR RA

Another area of research in RA is personalized medicine, which involves tailoring treatments to an individual's specific needs. With advancements in genetic testing, researchers have discovered that there are various subtypes of RA, which respond differently to various treatments. By identifying an individual's specific subtype of RA, doctors can develop more targeted treatment plans that are more likely to be effective. This approach has already been successful in treating other types of autoimmune disorders, such as multiple sclerosis.

THE ROLE OF TECHNOLOGY IN RA MANAGEMENT

Technology is also playing an increasingly important role in the management of RA. Wearable devices, such as activity trackers, can help patients monitor their activity levels and track their symptoms. Apps are also being developed to help patients keep track of their medications, log their symptoms, and get in touch with their healthcare providers. Telemedicine, which involves using video conferencing software to communicate with healthcare providers remotely, is becoming increasingly popular as a way for patients to receive care without having to leave their homes. This can be especially helpful for patients with limited mobility due to their RA.

CONCLUSION

While there is still no cure for rheumatoid arthritis, ongoing research is offering new hope for the millions of people around the world who live with this chronic condition. With advancements in personalized medicine, new drugs and treatments, and the use of technology to manage symptoms, the future of RA management looks promising.

Printed in Great Britain
by Amazon